AUTISM

Causes, Effects, and Diagnosis

Epris E. Ezekiel

Contents

The Background and Chronology of Autism

The official diagnosis of autism dates back to 1911. Paul Eugen Bleuler, a Swiss psychiatrist, came up with the word to refer to what he thought was schizophrenia in children.

Since then, we've learned more about autism, leading to the present diagnosis of autism spectrum disorder (ASD).

1920s: In the Monatsschrift für Psychiatrie und Neurologie (Monthly Journal of Psychiatry and Neurology), published in Kyiv, the Russian Empire, child psychiatrist Grunya Sukhareva describes six children who exhibit autistic characteristics.

1930s–1938: New York psychologist Louise Despert describes 29 childhood schizophrenia cases, some of which share characteristics with the current definition of autism.

1940s–1943: A report by Leo Kanner describes 11 patients who exhibited a "resistance to (unexpected) change" and were object-focused or preoccupied. Later on, he gave this illness the label "infantile autism."

1944: A case report detailing four children aged six to eleven is published by Hans Asperger, an Austrian doctor who received Nazi funding. Eugenics and the Nazi regime's "race hygiene" policies formed the basis of much of his science. He interprets the similar personalities or peculiarities of some of the children's parents as proof of a genetic connection. He served as a key figure in the creation of the phased-out functional categories (high vs. low functioning), and Asperger's syndrome, a former DSM diagnostic, bears his name.

1949: Kanner announces his notion that "refrigerator mothers," a word used to characterize chilly and aloof parents, are the cause of autism. This theory was refuted a long time ago.

1950s 1952: Children with autistic characteristics are classified as having childhood schizophrenia in the first edition of the Diagnostic and Statistical Manual of

Mental Disorders (DSM) published by the American Psychiatric Association.

In his study "The Autistic Child in Adolescence," published in 1956, Leon Eisenberg tracks 63 autistic children for nine years and then again at fifteen.

1959: Bruno Bettelheim, a physicist from Austria, writes about Joey, a 9-year-old autistic youngster, in Scientific American.

1960s: Bernard Rimland discusses the neurological components of autism and challenges the "refrigerator mother" explanation in his 1964 book Infantile Autism: The Syndrome and Its Implications for a Neural Explanation of Behavior.

1965: Children with autism are taught and cared for at the Sybil Elgar School.

The National Society of Autistic Children (now known as the Autism Society of America) was founded in 1965 by a group of allistic parents—those who are not on the autism spectrum—of autistic children.

Bruno Bettelheim's 1967 book The Empty Fortress: Infantile Autism and the Birth of the Self supports the idea that autism is caused by "refrigerator mothers."

Autism spectrum diseases are first proposed by psychiatrist Lorna Wing, MD, in the 1970s. She names the "triad of impairment," encompassing three domains: communication, imagination, and social interaction.

The Education for All Handicapped Children Act was passed in 1975. This act aimed to address the needs and safeguard the rights of children with impairments, the majority of whom had hitherto been denied access to education.

1977 saw the publication of the first study on twins and autism by Susan Folstein, MD, and Michael Rutter, MD. Genetics has a significant role in autism, according to the study.

The 1980s: The Diagnostic and Statistical Manual of Mental Disorders, Third Edition (DSM-III), incorporates criteria for diagnosing infantile autism for the first time.

1990s The Individuals with Disabilities Education Act (IDEA) added autism as a disability category in 1990, which made it simpler for autistic children to receive special education services.

Temple Grandin describes her life with autism and how she achieved success in her career in her 1996 book Emergence—Labeled Autistic.

1998: Measles, Mumps, and Rubella (MMR) vaccine may cause autism, according to a Lancet report by Andrew Wakefield, MBBS. After extensive epidemiological research disproves the theory, it is eventually withdrawn.

The Autism Awareness Puzzle Ribbon was adopted by the Autism Society in 1999 as "the universal sign of autism awareness." The autistic community now uses an infinity symbol (black or rainbow-colored) in place of the symbol since it implies that autistic individuals are incomplete and are linked to hate groups that target persons with autism.

The Global and Regional Asperger Syndrome Partnership (GRASP), an organization led by individuals with autism spectrum disorders including Asperger's syndrome, was established in the 2000s and 2003.

Stephen Edelson, PhD, and Bernard Rimland, MD, wrote the book Recovering Autistic Children in 2003.

2006: The Autistic Self Advocacy Network (ASAN) is founded by Ari Ne'eman.

In 2006, Dora Raymaker, PhD, and Christina Nicolaidis, MD, MP, established the Academic Autistic Spectrum Partnership in Research and Education (AASPIRE) to offer resources for autistic individuals and healthcare professionals.

2006: To fund autism research and treatment, the president signs the Combating Autism Act.

2010s: After the retraction of his study on autism, Andrew Wakefield is prohibited from practicing medicine and loses his medical license.

2013: Autism spectrum disorder is a combination of autism, Asperger's, and childhood disintegrative disorder according to the DSM-5.

2014: Reauthorizing and extending the Combating Autism Act, the president signs the Autism Collaboration, Accountability, Research, Education and Support (CARES) Act of 2014.

2016: One in 54 children has been diagnosed with autism spectrum disorder (ASD), according to the Centers for Disease Control and Prevention (CDC).

2020s: According to CDC projections, one out of every 36 children has been diagnosed with autism spectrum disorder (ASD).

2020: A comprehensive genetic sequencing study finds 102 genes linked to autism that are crucial in forming the early brain.

These historical occurrences continue to inform autism research and advocacy. The goal of autistic self-advocates is to advance a future in which autistic individuals are fully accepted and understood, as they gain more public recognition and political clout.

Additionally, advocates strive to make resources accessible to fill the support gaps that autistic adults and children currently face.

Chapter 1

What's Autism?

Autism spectrum disorder (ASD), another name for autism, is a complicated developmental illness that impacts a person's behavior, learning, interaction, and communication. Differences in brain function among people with ASD may affect their social interactions and behavior.

Autism manifests before the age of three and lasts the entirety of a person's life. As a spectrum condition, it impacts individuals differently and to differing degrees.

Autistic people may struggle with:

- ❖ **Sensational arousal.** They also differ in their responses to various stimuli, including temperature, sound, light, and clothing. An intense, excessively focused interest in subjects or activities is another typical indication of ASD. The number of youngsters receiving an autism diagnosis has increased. Yet, rather than more children having the illness, the most recent figures may be higher due to greater awareness and modifications in the diagnosis process. Researchers continue to learn more about the interplay of biological, environmental, and genetic components in ASD.

People with autism may be diagnosed as adults even though they have had the disorder since they were young. It can occur when the symptoms of autism are not severe enough to interfere with day-to-day functioning.

For children with ASD, early intervention promotes better development, which may facilitate day-to-day functioning as an adult.

- ❖ **Changes.** Changes in daily routine and transitions can be difficult for people with autism.
- ❖ **Studying.** Learning difficulties, such as a delayed rate of skill development, can

accompany autism. A person with autism, for instance, might struggle with communication but excel in art, music, math, or memory-related tasks. As a result, they may perform particularly well on analytical or problem-solving tests.

❖ **Communication.** Someone with autism may have trouble communicating and comprehending the feelings and thoughts of others. As a result, they find it challenging to communicate through touch, facial expressions, and words or gestures.

Labels for Autism Functions

Everybody with autism is affected differently. The phrases "high-functioning" and "low-functioning" are occasionally used to characterize autism. However, some people may find these labels offensive.

Even though these labels are not medical words, people still frequently use them informally to characterize autism.

Describe low-functioning autism.

An intellectual handicap affects about 30% of individuals with autism. This indicates that they occasionally can't live alone and may require assistance with daily duties. This is commonly referred to as "low-functioning autism."

What is autism with high functioning?

There may be others with autism who have less overt symptoms. They frequently perform well academically and have fewer communication issues. The most common names for this are "high-functioning autism" or the antiquated "Asperger syndrome."

The DSM-5, a guide used by medical professionals to identify mental illnesses, now includes three ASD severity categories added by the American Psychiatric Association (APA). These levels outline the degree of assistance required for an individual with autism based on their social communication requirements and behaviors:

Level 1: Mild, in need of assistance

Level 2: Moderate, needing significant (or significant) assistance

Level 3: Extreme, necessitating significant assistance

When discussing the impact of autism, you can use phrases like "more significant" or "less significant." Even better, find out from an autistic person or their caregiver how they would like to characterize their condition.

Symptoms of Autism

Autism symptoms typically start to show before a child turns three. Some exhibit symptoms from birth.

✓ Problems adjusting to routine
✓ Speaking with a flat, robotic, or sing-song voice

- ✓ Issues with facial expressions, tone of voice, gestures, or speech comprehension or use
- ✓ Not wishing to be hugged or held

- ✓ Not paying attention when someone else calls your attention to something
- ✓ Ignoring and not paying attention to others
- ✓ Extremely sensitive to sensations, noises, scents, or sights that others might consider normal
- ✓ Repeating words or phrases, rocking back and forth, or fussing with things (such as switching a light switch) are repetitive behaviors.
- ✓ A limited variety of interests or a strong passion for particular subjects
- ✓ Absence of eye contact

Seizures can also occur in some autistic individuals. Perhaps these won't begin till adolescence.

Adults with autism symptoms

Adults with autism may exhibit some symptoms. Typical signs and symptoms may include:

- ✓ Being unintentionally direct, uninterested, or impolite to others
- ✓ Taking things literally or failing to recognize sarcasm
- ✓ Having trouble putting your feelings into words
- ✓ Maintaining everyday routines and being agitated when they vary
- ✓ Fear of social situations
- ✓ Deciding to live alone or struggling to make friends
- ✓ Having trouble figuring out what other people are feeling or thinking

Adults with autism may also exhibit the following symptoms:

- ✓ Desiring to meticulously prepare things before executing them
- ✓ Recognizing patterns, noises, smells, or minute nuances that others miss
- ✓ Having a strong interest in certain things
- ✓ Getting too close to people or becoming angry if they touch you or get too close
- ✓ Lack of awareness of social cues or "rules"

✓ Not making eye contact.

Children with autism symptoms

Autism in children can manifest in a variety of ways. They could consist of:

✓ Fear of things, either more or less than one may often anticipate

✓ Unusual eating or sleeping patterns

✓ Cognitive, linguistic, motor, or learning delays

✓ Flails their hands, spin in circles, or rock their body.

✓ Displays compulsive hobbies

✓ Arrange toys in a particular arrangement and become agitated if it is altered.

✓ Doesn't act, dance, or sing for you by the age of sixty months

✓ Is 36 months old and doesn't notice or desire to play with other kids.

✓ Is 24 months old and unable to comprehend

when others are upset or depressed.

- ✓ By the time they are 12 months old, they are not using motions like saying hi.
- ✓ By the age of twelve months, they no longer wish to play basic games like pat-a-cake.
- ✓ Nine months old and incapable of displaying facial expressions
- ✓ By nine months old, they are not responding to their name.

Stimming

Hand and arm flapping, rocking, spinning, twirling, bouncing, head-banging, and other similar body movements are examples of self-stimulating behaviors, or "stimming." A rubber band flicking, a thread twirling, touching something with a particular texture, and other repetitive actions can also be included.

For amusement, to relieve boredom, or as a coping mechanism for stress or anxiety, people with autism may stim. They may be able to modify the amount of sensory input with its assistance. To tune out a loud or distressing noise, kids can, for instance, twist a string to observe it or concentrate on a single sound.

Sometimes a situation can overwhelm an autistic person, leaving them unable to react appropriately. They may have a breakdown as a result. More than just a tantrum, a meltdown is an uncontrollable nervous system reaction in an autistic individual. They might shout, cry, or physically act out by biting, striking, or kicking. They can fully shut down and cease to react at all. The body's physical reaction to an intense emotional or sensory experience is known as a meltdown.

When someone with autism is having a meltdown, make sure they are in a safe place, give them space, and treat them with respect.

Chapter 2

Different forms of autism

Previously, doctors believed that autism or related developmental problems might be divided into several categories. Since the conditions listed below are included in the spectrum of autistic disorders, they are no longer used:

- **Widespread developmental disease (atypical autism or PDD).** If your child exhibits certain autistic behaviors, such as impairments in social and communication skills, but does not fall into another category, your doctor may use this phrase.

- **Disintegrative condition in children.** Children with this disease develop normally for at least two years before losing some or most of their social and communicative skills.

- **Autism.** This is what most people think of when

they hear the term "autism." It impacts children under three years old's play, social connections, and communication.

❖ **Asperger's syndrome.** Regarding intelligence testing, children with Asperger syndrome typically score in the average or higher range. However, their interests may be limited and they may struggle with social skills.

What Leads to Autism?

It's unclear exactly why autism occurs. It might be caused by issues with the areas of your brain that process language and interpret sensory information.

People of any race, nationality, or social background can develop autism. A child's likelihood of developing autism is unaffected by family income, lifestyle, or educational attainment. However, a few risk factors are as follows:

✓ Having elderly parents as parents
✓ Being a man or having been born a man.

- ✓ The prevalence of autism is four times higher in boys than in girls.
- ✓ A sibling who has autism
- ✓ Genetic disorders such as Down syndrome, Rett, and fragile X
- ✓ Incredibly low birth weight

Does autism have a hereditary component? Specific gene combinations may increase a child's risk because autism runs in families. Autism may be caused by changes in over 1,000 genes. However, not all of them have expert confirmation. Between 40% and 80% of an individual's risk of autism can be influenced by genetic factors.

Your overall risk is determined by the combination of your genes, environment, parents' ages, and any birth defects.

About 2% to 4% of individuals with autism are likely to have an uncommon gene mutation or chromosome problem as their only cause. This typically occurs in disorders, such as mutations in the ADNP gene, affecting other body sections. A person with ADNP syndrome will have particular facial features in addition to autism symptoms.

There are numerous genes linked to brain development that are implicated in autism. This could explain why sociability, cognitive functioning, and communication problems are common among autistic symptoms.

Potential Pregnancy Risk Factors for Autism
Other theories on potential risk factors for autism during pregnancy exist in addition to the known risk factors. It's uncertain if these characteristics are probable causes of autism, even if research has shown a link between them.

Vitamin insufficiency in pregnancy
A 2020 study that assessed iron deficiencies during pregnancy discovered a correlation between increased autism risks and decreased iron intakes.7 Prenatal iron shortage is unlikely to be a risk factor for autism on its

own because low maternal iron is linked to neurological development and other brain development issues. However, consuming enough iron during pregnancy is a straightforward method to safeguard the developing brain of your fetus.

Furthermore, taking folic acid, the synthetic form of folate, in the early stages of pregnancy considerably reduces the incidence of autism, according to a 2022 meta-analysis of ten research.8 A lower risk of autism was linked to taking 400 micrograms (mcg) of folic acid.

Everyone capable of becoming pregnant, including those who are not attempting to conceive, should consume 400–800 micrograms of folate or folic acid per day. Fortified foods like bread and cereal provide the majority of people with approximately 150 mcg of folic acid per day.

Contamination of the air

Air pollution exposure during all three trimesters of pregnancy raised the incidence of ASD, according to a

2022 study, particularly for kids born with a male gender assignment. However, once more, experts view this as a risk factor in vulnerable populations rather than a danger factor on its own.

According to M. Daniele Fallin, Ph.D., director of the Wendy Klag Center for Autism and Developmental Disabilities at the Johns Hopkins Bloomberg School of Public Health, "information regarding environmental risk during pregnancy is really at its infancy, so any data-supported hypotheses must be investigated further as nothing is yet considered a certain cause." Expectant mothers need to take proactive, safe measures that may help protect their unborn children.

To protect oneself from air pollution, the American Lung Association suggests several measures. For instance, when pollution levels are high, exercise indoors, avoid busy locations, and fill up your petrol tank after dark. The U.S. Air Quality Index is available on the Environmental Protection Agency's Air Now website, where you may see the daily air quality values in your location.

Gaining weight during pregnancy

High body mass index (BMI) and excessive pregnancy weight increase were linked to the children's risk of ASD, according to a 2020 systematic study. Scientists hypothesize that hormone dysregulation linked to excessive weight gain may impact embryonic brain development.

According to Anna Maria Wilms Floet, M.D., a behavioral developmental pediatrician at the Kennedy Krieger Institute's Center for Autism and Related Disorders in Baltimore, "the prevalence of obesity and autism has increased over the past few decades, but that does not imply that the two are related."

Nevertheless, you might get the finest pregnancy results if you follow the suggested weight increase guidelines.

Chapter 3

Testing for Autism

Obtaining a definitive diagnosis of autism can be challenging. Your physician will concentrate on development and behavior.

Diagnosing children typically involves two phases.

- ➢ Should these tests reveal any indications of a problem, your child will require a more thorough assessment. Without a doctor's referral, you can still ask your state's early intervention office for an autism evaluation for your child. A qualified professional, frequently a developmental-behavioral pediatrician or child psychologist, will examine a variety of factors to determine whether your kid has autism.

You will be questioned extensively by the professional regarding the behavior, communication, and growth of your child. Additionally, they will assess your child's cognitive, verbal, and self-help skills (feeding, dressing, and using the restroom) using several tests. Your child's behavior will be observed by the specialist. Your child's symptoms and your concerns may also lead an occupational therapist and speech-language pathologist to evaluate them.

Additionally, your doctor might suggest genetic testing or exams for hearing and vision. These elements aid the team in arriving at an accurate diagnosis.

> A developmental screening will let your doctor know if your kid is progressing as expected in areas like speech, behavior, learning, and movement. Doctors should screen for these developmental deficits around the age of nine, eighteen, twenty-four, or thirty months, according to experts. During the 18-month and 24-month checks, pediatricians regularly do specialized autism screening on youngsters.

What to do following a diagnosis of autism

To feel your best after receiving a diagnosis of autism, follow these steps:

Be mindful of additional health concerns.

Even while autism is not a disease, many autistic people may also have other diseases like dyslexia, ADHD, and others. Talk to your doctor about any concerns you may have regarding your health or the health of your kid.

Obtain the assistance you require.

Seek support if you or your kid feel isolated after receiving an autism diagnosis. You can manage a diagnosis with the help of national advocacy groups, support groups, your doctor, other autistic people on social media, or your school, workplace, or college.

Pay attention to those with autism.

To learn more about the disease, you can use a variety of blogs, books, and videos. You can learn more about autism by listening to people with the condition tell their stories.

Finish your homework.

Autism articles are available for you to read. Although there is a wealth of information available, you only need to consult a few reliable sites to begin learning about your diagnosis.

Give yourself enough time to comprehend the diagnosis.

You may experience a variety of feelings. Be aware that you can ask your doctor for assistance. Even after receiving a diagnosis, you can carry on with your regular life.

Chapter 4

What Kinds of Therapies Are Effective for Autism?

Numerous therapies can assist individuals with autism develop their skills and lessen their symptoms. The likelihood of your child succeeding is increased if you begin therapy early, such as during preschool or earlier, but it's never too late to get help.

The American Academy of Pediatrics (AAP) advises against waiting for a formal diagnosis of autism and to begin looking into therapy as soon as you suspect your kid has the disorder. To receive a formal diagnosis, some tests, follow-ups with specialists, and time may be required.

What works for each individual is different. Learn about a few of the most well-liked and effective remedies.

Engaging in Play Therapy

Compared to ordinary children, children with autism frequently play differently. Instead of concentrating on the entire toy, they will probably concentrate on its components, such as its wheels. Like other children, they "pretend to play." They might also be reluctant to play with other people.

However, for many kids with autism spectrum disorder (ASD), playing is their means of self-expression; their motions and toys can serve as their speech. Children with ASD can learn and connect with other kids and adults in a way that makes sense to them through play.

Play therapy can help children think more creatively, develop their language or communication skills, enhance their social and emotional abilities, and broaden their toy play and interpersonal relationships.

Any of the following types of play therapy can help children with ASD:

IPGs, or integrated play groups.

Children with and without autism spectrum conditions are combined so that the former can learn how to play and follow the example of their peers. There are just a few kids with ASD in each group, which consists of three to   five   kids.

The youngsters eventually take over the play, but the adults set the tone. As your child engages in IPGs, they may eventually engage in more role play and have several opportunities to develop their social skills while interacting with other children.

IPGs can meet for up to 3 hours a week. Research reveals that children with ASD who received two 30-minute IPG sessions a week for 4 months increased their quality of play, used their toys in a more usual fashion, and demonstrated improved social engagement with their peers.

One popular kind of play therapy is floortime. To play with your child on their terms, you, a teacher, or a therapist get down on the floor. You participate by playing the game in the same manner as your child, then you add a new element.

To add language to the game, it may be a few words or a second toy. In order to promote greater communication and give your child's play something new, the idea is to design play that alternates between you and them. They should learn how to better focus their thoughts and develop emotionally as a result.

For Floortime, your child can spend up to 25 hours a week with a therapist, or you and your child can do it at home. According to studies, the majority of kids who receive 25 hours a week of floortime therapy for two years or more see improvements in every developmental domain.

JASPER stands for joint attention, symbolic play engagement, and regulation.

can improve your child's ability to focus on both a person and a toy simultaneously. Their ability to play with other kids can be enhanced by developing joint attention abilities. Additionally, the JASPER program can help your child develop other social skills, widen their toy play, talk to people more, and play pretend more.

Children undergoing JASPER therapy frequently receive one-on-one sessions with a therapist. In preschool settings, JASPER is occasionally available. Children can receive up to 25 hours of this kind of therapy each week.

Within a few weeks, you might observe that your youngster learns new skills. As they play, they may be talking more. Or rather than merely spinning the wheels, they might be "driving" cars down a ramp. Depending on their needs, this kind of therapy could last for months or years.

Occupational Therapy

Activities of daily living and the usage of commonplace items, such as learning how to button a shirt or hold a fork correctly, are assisted by occupational therapy. But anything that has to do with job, school, or recreation can be included. The needs and objectives of the kid determine the focus.

What is the job of an occupational therapist?

Occupational therapists collaborate with other professionals, such as teachers and parents. They assist in establishing clear objectives for the autistic individual. These objectives frequently touch on conduct, classroom performance, and social interaction.

Evaluation and therapy are the two primary ways that occupational therapists can assist.

The therapist observes children to see whether they are capable of performing activities that are appropriate for their age, such as dressing or playing a game. To see how the child interacts with others and objects in their environment, the therapist may occasionally have the child videotaped throughout the day. This aids the therapist in figuring out what kind of care the youngster requires. The therapist may examine in detail:

- ✓ The way the kid and caretakers interact
- ✓ A variety of actions, including aggression
- ✓ Reactions to various stimuli, such as touch
- ✓ The necessity of personal space
- ✓ Use your play talents.
- ✓ Make the switch to a new activity

✓ The capacity for sustained attention and endurance

After gathering data, an occupational therapist can create a plan for your kid. There is no one perfect course of treatment. However, early, systematic, customized therapy is most effective.

Many concepts can be combined in occupational therapy, such as:

✓ Adaptive techniques, such as undergoing changes
✓ Activities for development, such as combing hair and cleaning teeth
✓ Play activities that promote communication and interaction

Engaging in physical hobbies such as bead stringing or puzzle solving can help children develop body awareness and coordination.

What are the advantages of occupational therapy

for individuals with ASD?

Helping individuals with autism enhance their quality of life at home and at school is the main objective of occupational therapy. To help persons with autism become as autonomous as possible, the therapist helps them learn, maintain, and enhance skills.

Occupational therapy could be useful for:

- ✓ Play, self-care, communication, social skills, and problem-solving
- ✓ Visual literacy for writing and reading
- ✓ Knowledge of their body and how it relates to other people
- ✓ Perceptual abilities such as recognizing color, shape, and size differences, sitting, or posture
- ✓ Toilet training, clothing, tooth brushing, and other personal hygiene abilities are examples of everyday living skills.
- ✓ The ability to grasp objects in their hands while writing or using scissors requires fine motor abilities.

✓ The gross motor skills required for riding a bike, walking, and climbing stairs

Occupational therapy can help a child with autism develop these abilities:

✓ Develop self-control.

✓ Play with other kids.

✓ Use more suitable language while expressing your emotions.

✓ Develop the ability to postpone gratification.

Speech Therapy

Significant issues with speech and nonverbal communication can be present in those with ASD. They could also have an extremely difficult time socializing. For these reasons, a key component of autism treatment is speech therapy. It facilitates speaking, communication, and social interaction in kids. It may entail nonverbal communication abilities such as maintaining eye contact, sharing the discourse, and utilizing and comprehending gestures. Additionally, children may learn how to communicate through computers, sign language, or image symbols.

Chapter 5

Which speech and communication problems are typical among people with autism?

In order to properly communicate with others, one in three individuals with autism struggle to make speech sounds.

An autistic person may:

- ✓ Employ appropriate sentences and phrases, but speak in an uninspiring manner.
- ✓ Echolalia is the practice of parrots or people who frequently repeat what others have said.
- ✓ Use "words" that seem strange or speak robotically.

- ✓ Talk incoherently using word-like sounds
- ✓ Not a word
- ✓ Talk or hum melodically.
- ✓ Screams, yells, groans, or harsh, throaty noises

Additionally, a person with autism may struggle with communicating in ways like:

- ✓ Absence of imaginative language
- ✓ Insufficient comprehension of the meaning of symbols or words
- ✓ Echolalia, or repeating someone else's words while they are being said, is the primary method of communication.
- ✓ Memorizing what has been heard without understanding what has been stated
- ✓ Having trouble understanding words that were acquired in a different context
- ✓ Difficulties with eye contact and gestures in talking

Learning to talk is not enough for a youngster with autism. Additionally, the child needs to learn how to communicate through language. That entails being able to carry on a discussion. It also entails being aware of other people's body language, tone of voice, and facial expressions in addition to their spoken words.

How does speech therapy fit into the autism treatment process?

Therapists who specialize in treating speech impairments and language issues are known as speech-language pathologists. They play a crucial role in the team that treats autism. When it comes to diagnosing autism and referring patients to other specialists, speech therapists frequently take the lead in early screening and detection.

Following a diagnosis of autism, speech therapists determine the most effective strategies to enhance communication. In close collaboration with the family, school, and other experts, the speech-language pathologist works. The following speech alternatives may be introduced by the speech therapist if the autistic person is nonverbal or has significant speech difficulties:

- ✓ Singing melodies that correspond with the sentences' rhythm, intensity, and flow
- ✓ Teaching children to communicate through the use of visuals rather than words
- ✓ Improving speech articulation through lip massage or face muscle exercise
- ✓ Computerized "talkers"
- ✓ Typing or signing

Research backs up some of these techniques more than it does others. Make sure to go over them in detail with both your child's pediatrician and the speech-language pathologist.

What are the advantages of speech therapy for those with ASD?

Communication in general can be enhanced with speech therapy. This enables individuals with autism to enhance their capacity to build relationships and carry out daily tasks.

One of speech therapy's specific objectives is to assist the person with autism:

- ✓ Develop self-control.
- ✓ Take pleasure in conversing, playing, and engaging with others.
- ✓ Use communication techniques to build relationships.
- ✓ Share your thoughts.
- ✓ Develop your ability to converse
- ✓ Engage in conversation without waiting for others to initiate it.
- ✓ Recognize how individuals communicate both verbally and nonverbally, and know what they mean in various contexts.
- ✓ Use both verbal and nonverbal communication.
- ✓ Use clear, concise language

For autism, when is the ideal time to begin speech therapy?

Speech treatment should begin as soon as possible.

Typically, autism spectrum condition is evident before the age of three. It is possible to identify language delays as early as 18 months of age. Some people with autism can be diagnosed as early as 10 to 12 months of age. Speech therapy can have the greatest impact if initiated as soon as possible.

When diagnosed and treated early, two out of three preschool-aged autistic children improve their spoken language comprehension and communication abilities. Research shows that those who receive the most speech treatment tends to progress the most.

Analysis of Applied Behavior (ABA)

Rewards are used in this kind of therapy to teach new skills and reinforce positive habits. To provide the autistic child with moment-by-moment input, parents and other caregivers undergo training.

The individual determines the aims of treatment, which could include schoolwork, social skills, communication, and personal hygiene. Studies show that children who receive early, rigorous ABA can make significant, long-lasting improvements.

Different forms of ABA exist. Among them are:

- ❖ **PRT, or pivotal response therapy.** Important aspects of a child's development, such as self-control and taking the initiative in social settings, are highlighted here.
- ❖ **Intervention for verbal behavior (VBI).** The aim is to enhance a child's verbal abilities.
- ❖ **DTT stands for discrete trial training.** This simplifies a desired action into its most basic components.
- ❖ **EIBI stands for early intensive behavioral**

intervention. Young children, typically under five, are the target audience for this type of ABA.

Chapter 6

Autism and Diets

Autism is a complicated neurological condition. There is no concrete proof that specific diets benefit kids with ASD. Before trying something new, like a specific diet, see your doctor.

Some autistic kids may seem like finicky eaters. They might consume more or less food, only foods with a particular color or texture, or non-food items. They may experience constipation, which causes them to feel full when they are not, or they may cough or gag during meals.

Although eliminating some foods can seem to help your child's symptoms, it might have the opposite effect.

For instance, the bones of children with autism are frequently thinner. Dairy products include nutrients that can strengthen bones. Research on casein, a protein found in milk products, has shown that many kids behaved similarly whether or not they consumed foods containing this protein. Their autism symptoms didn't significantly alter.

However, some dietary adjustments might help with specific autistic symptoms. For example, dietary sensitivities may exacerbate behavioral issues. Taking the allergen out of your child's diet could help with some behavioral problems.

What matters is that the food your child eats should support both their unique nutritional requirements and the symptoms of ASD. The best method to choose the most beneficial diet is to consult a nutrition specialist, such as a registered dietitian, and your physician. They'll assist you in creating a kid-friendly meal plan.

Digestive issues such as nausea, vomiting, or constipation might affect some kids with autism. A diet recommended by your physician won't exacerbate these problems.

Autism supplements

There is evidence to suggest that some vitamins and minerals may be deficient in individuals with autism.

Autism spectrum disorder is not brought on by this. However, to boost nutrition, your doctor could recommend vitamins. Among the supplements most frequently prescribed to individuals with autism are vitamin B and magnesium. However, consumers should avoid taking megavitamins because they can cause overdosing.

Additionally, keep in mind that dietary requirements vary over time. As your kid grows older, the dietitian will assist you in ensuring that the foods they consume continue to match their nutritional needs.

Chapter 7

How to Support Your Autistic Child

Communication

You can improve your child's communication if they have autism by:

- ✓ Making eye contact, using simple gestures, or using illustrations to help them grasp what you're saying

- ✓ Allowing them more time to process what you just stated

- ✓ Using basic, unambiguous language

- ✓ Speaking clearly and slowly

- ✓ To let them know you're talking to them, use their name.

Refrain from:

- ✓ Asking a lot of questions to your child

- ✓ Conversing in a busy or noisy setting

- ✓ Saying phrases like "break a leg" have multiple meanings.

Having trouble falling asleep

Many children with autism struggle to get to sleep and stay asleep. You can assist them by:

- ✓ Speaking with a physician about problems that could interfere with their sleep
- ✓ Maintaining a quiet and dark bedroom
- ✓ Allowing them to sleep with earplugs if they are helpful
- ✓ Observing the same nightly nighttime routine
- ✓ Maintaining a sleep log to identify common problems

Socializing

To encourage your youngster to socialize and form friendships:

- ✓ Seek out or peruse information from other parents of autistic children.
- ✓ To find local social groups that can support people with autism, check out the National

Autism Society directory.

- ✓ Seek advice from your autism care team.
- ✓ Find out if your child's school can assist.

Be careful not to:

- ✓ Put your child under strain. Allow them to develop social skills over time.
- ✓ If your child prefers to be alone, push them into social situations.

Disparities in Autism

Different groups of people are affected by autism in different ways. Additionally, this can occasionally result in unequal access to assistance, diagnosis, and treatment. To guarantee that everyone has equal access to autism care, regardless of gender, color, or sexual orientation, it is critical to comprehend autism inequalities or differences.

Women with autism

Women's autism can occasionally differ from men's. In contrast to men, cisgender women with autism may:

- ✓ Try to "fit in" by imitating others without autism or by hiding symptoms of the disorder.
- ✓ Be quieter

- ✓ Keep their emotions hidden.
- ✓ Reduce the occurrence of recurrent behaviors
- ✓ Appear to handle social settings more adeptly.

Your doctor may be less experienced in diagnosing autism in women and girls. It can be more difficult to determine whether a girl or woman has autism because many of the symptoms are exclusive to men with the disorder. As a result, girls and women with autism may go undiagnosed or be completely overlooked. The estimates of the proportion of men with autism compared to women have decreased as professionals have become more aware of this.

Final Thought

ASD, often known as autism spectrum disorder, is a complicated developmental brain condition that impacts social relationships, behavior, learning, and communication. Autism is diagnosed at any age; however, it manifests before the age of three. The impact of ASD varies from person to person, as does its severity. Although there is no known cure for autism, persons with the disorder can manage difficult symptoms and lead fulfilling lives with the support of developmental, behavioral, and speech therapies, such as applied behavior analysis (ABA), and early intervention. Consult your physician to find out the next steps for screening, diagnosis, and assistance if you have concerns about your child's development or your symptoms.

9 798304 675666